HOPE

September 2019

Brain Injury
HOPE
MAGAZINE
*"Supporting the
Brain Injury Community"*

Welcome

HOPE MAGAZINE

Serving the Brain Injury Community Since 2015

September 2019

Publisher
David A. Grant

Editor
Sarah Grant

Our Contributors

Patrick Brigham
Rachel Dombeck
Debra Gorman
Regina Káró
Kelly Lang
Elizabeth Peirce
Andrea Rauser
James Scott

Welcome to the September 2019 issue of HOPE Magazine

For those of us who live daily as part of the brain injury community, we've learned that life is all about change.

Brain injury does indeed change everything. Family dynamics change. Some people walk out of our lives – never to be seen again, while new and cherished friendships emerge. Relationships take on new form, some end in pain, while others are made stronger by circumstance – and certainly not choice.

No one asks for brain injury to be part of life.

In this month's issue of HOPE Magazine, you'll see some changes. Rest easy, as you will find the types of stories that have inspired our readers for years. You will, however, see change in how we present HOPE Magazine.

This is an "us" publication. If you see something you like – or something you don't – we would love to hear from you. Every opinion matters.

Peace to all who live lives affected by brain injury.

David A. Grant
Publisher

Contents

ON THE COVER

Sunflowers, a symbol of hope and growth are a fitting choice for our late summer issue.

QUOTABLE

"I am not my brain injury. I am a person who sustained a brain injury. I am a person first!"

SAVE THE DATE

November 22, 2019
Krempels Center Craft Fair
Portsmouth, NH
Learn more at
www.krempelscenter.org

You Look Fine

By Kelly Lang

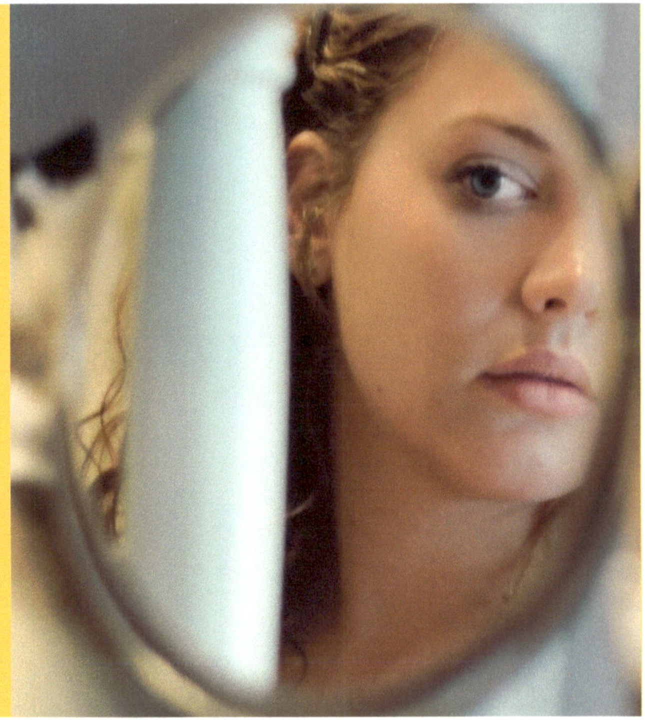

You look fine! If only I had a dollar for every time I have heard those three words. Of course, I am thrilled my daughter doesn't have scars or other physical signs following her traumatic brain injury. Surprisingly, looking fine has become an issue.

Olivia's injury is the result of a horrific motor vehicle accident in November 2001 when she was just three years old. She was not expected to survive. Her pediatric neurologist called her a "miracle child." After reviewing the MRI, he commented to me he had seen many brain injuries over the years and hers was catastrophic. He worked with patients who had less severe injuries and never learned to eat, walk, or talk again. She has learned all those things and more.

She does not remember her "before." This, too, is both a curse and a blessing. At three, she started attending preschool two mornings a week and loved to play with figurines and Barbies. She was only learning her letters and the concept of sharing. She doesn't have any memory of those times. I am not sure if it's due to the injury or the fact she was only three.

> *"Issues began once she reached first grade and her learning difficulties became more apparent. Her processing issues slowed her down and the social issues started escalating."*

While in kindergarten, following two years in the special education preschool, Olivia did not stand out amongst her classmates. She was in a program for kindergartners who needed a bit of extra help learning, but other than that she fit in. Issues began once she reached first grade and her learning difficulties became more apparent. Her processing issues slowed her down and the social issues started escalating. As the years went on these issues would continue and, in some cases, get worse before any improvement.

I always made a point to meet with her teachers prior to the beginning of the school year for the purpose of explaining why she had an Individualized Education Plan (IEP), and how her disability affected her. A number of these teachers and case managers approached me during the year and commented how helpful the information was since she walked into the classroom trying to blend in as much as possible. Once they got to know her, the issues became more apparent.

She graduated from high school in June 2017. This was a huge accomplishment. She has taken a few classes at the local community college and many of her professors have asked her why she has accommodations. We had to meet with the Director of Disability Services and after Olivia left to get to class the Director said, "WOW, she can communicate well." Stunner, I didn't even have a response. I walked out incredulous that the Director of Disability Services would make that comment, especially to a parent.

Unfortunately, the invisible disability has been a detriment to Olivia over and over. Peers have a difficult time communicating with her because she cannot process the information. She becomes forgetful and doesn't respond to messages, she will not be able to drive, she is fearful of loud noises, etc. I could go on and on.

When a doctor or therapist comments about her "looking fine," I understandably become very upset. These are the "experts" and I need them to understand her ability and disability. I realize they only see her for a fraction of her day, and she is on her best behavior.

Always eager to make a good impression, I need them to listen closely for the clues that indicate she is not fine. She is struggling and her family is struggling alongside of her.

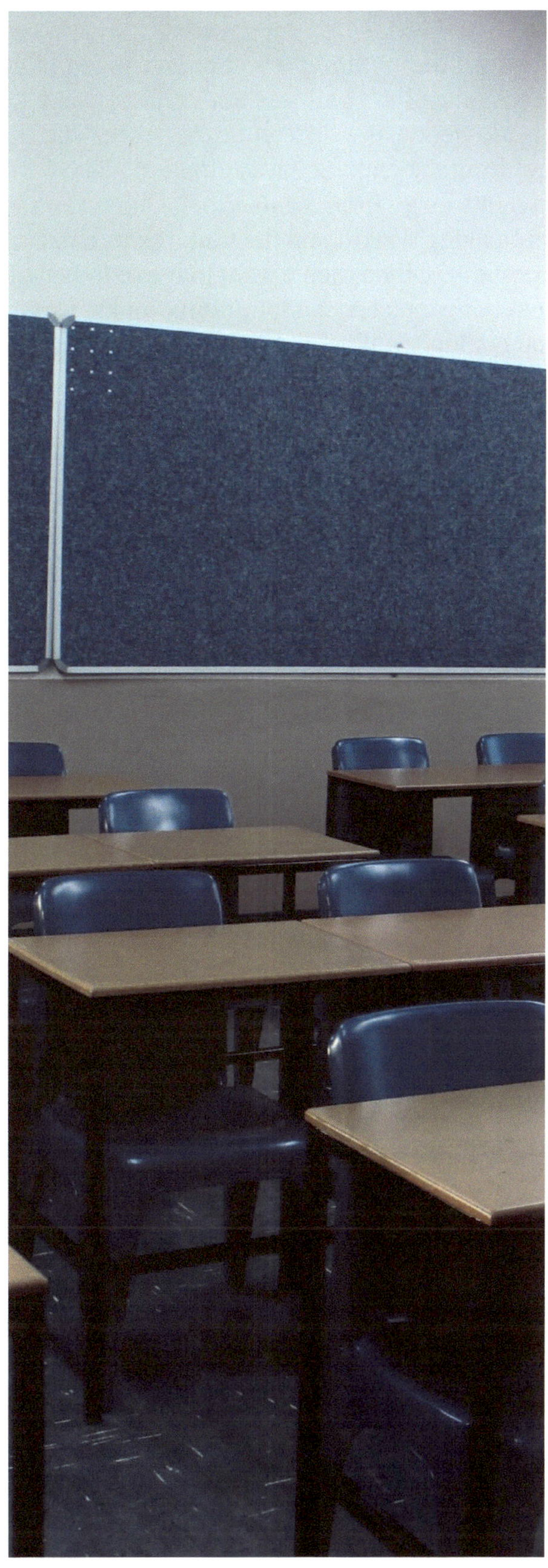

During a recent family vacation, we hiked in the Smoky Mountains. The climb to a waterfall was beautiful and the trail was not very crowded. Olivia does not function well when there are crowds. The descent was a different experience. The trail dropped off a bit to the right if you walked a few feet from the path. She was afraid to walk. I walked on the right side giving her more room to navigate away from the drop off. Our system was working really well until another hiker or group came along walking up the trail. It was narrow and only allowed two or four people, depending on the width. Olivia didn't want to move to her right for fear of falling down the cliff and I would try to help but we received a lot of dirty looks. I wished we had something to indicate she has a disability and couldn't walk securely.

I am eternally grateful Olivia did not suffer any noticeable physical impairments. There are some but not any visible to someone who does not know her well. My goal is to educate others about brain injury and the effects it has on the survivor as well as the family. I hope others will learn things are not always as they seem.

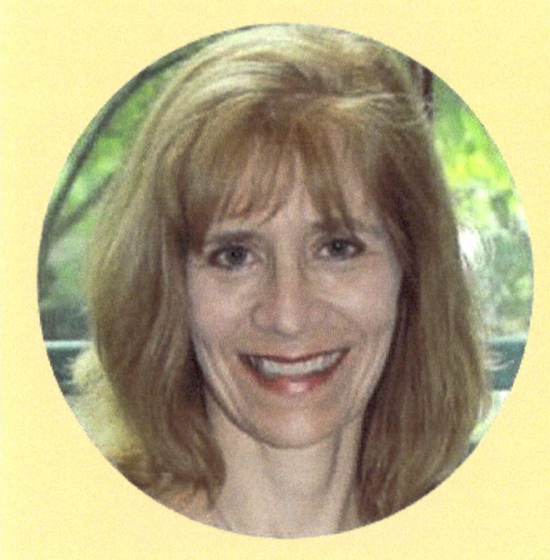

Meet Kelly Lang

Kelly Lang and her family live in Northern Virginia. Kelly's advocacy career began once Olivia arrived in the acute care setting and has continued for the past seventeen years. Kelly has served on the Board of the Brain Injury Association of Virginia since 2012 and has been a member of the Brain Injury Association of America's Brain Injury Council since 2016. Kelly's daughter, Olivia, was profiled in the Brain Injury Association of America's poster campaign in 2006. Olivia was the first pediatric speaker at the Brain Injury Congressional Task Force Panel in March 2017. Kelly can be found through her website at TheMiracleChild.org.

Living With Hope

By Patrick Brigham

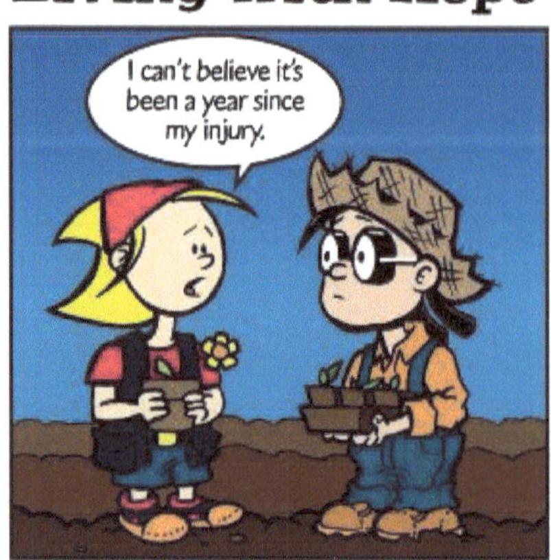

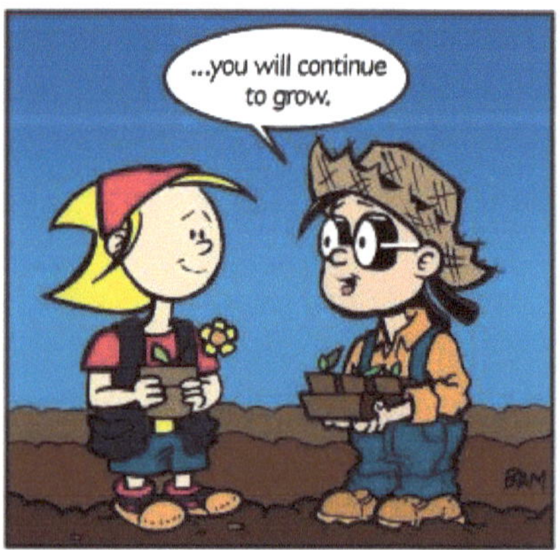

Contributors Wanted
Share Your Story in HOPE Magazine

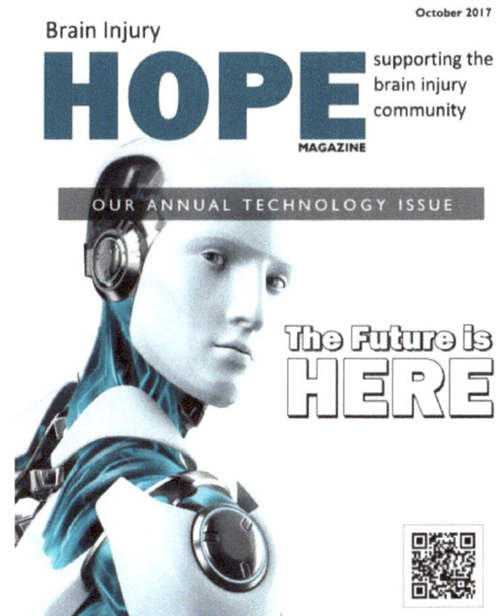

Do you have a story that you'd like to share with the world? If so, we'd love to hear from you! HOPE Magazine is always looking for stories to publish in our monthly magazine.

It doesn't matter whether you are a survivor, caregiver, family member or part of the professional or support community. We ALL have something to offer!

Your Story Has Value

- ▶ We prefer an article length of 800-1,000 words. Longer or shorter pieces will be considered.
- ▶ When submitting, please include a photo or photos to be included with your piece.
- ▶ We happily offer a link back to your blog, website, or most anywhere pertinent.
- ▶ Please include a short biography, preferably under 150 words.
- ▶ Please include 2-3 photos to accompany your submission
- ▶ Previously published pieces are acceptable for submission. Just let us know where your piece was previously published.
- ▶ Any topic that resonates within the brain injury/concussion community will be considered.
- ▶ Submissions that directly or indirectly promote a specific product, or business will be rejected.
- ▶ Submissions need to either be in Microsoft Word or in Notepad format. PDF's and links to content posted on an existing website will not be considered for publication.

Submission is Easy. Email Your Story to: mystory@tbihopeandinspiration.com

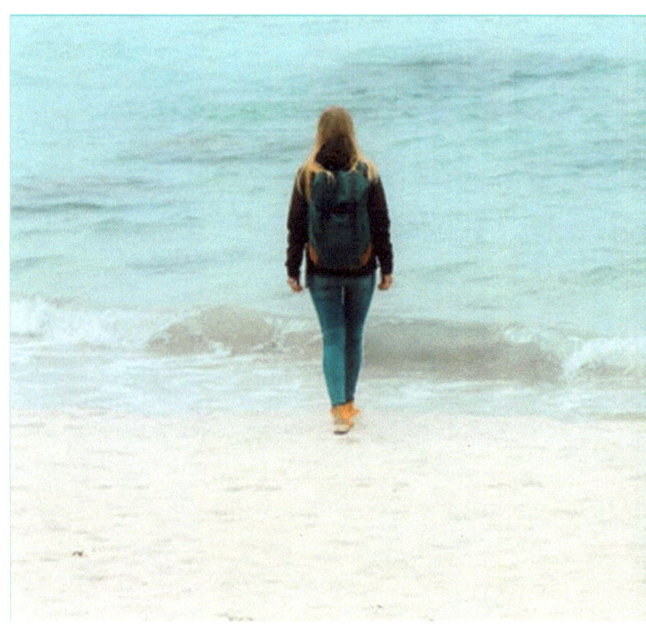

Recovering Your Spirit

By Elizabeth Peirce

What I remember most is the sound of my head hitting the polished hardwood floor of the gym, and thinking, "Wow, that sounded just like a bowling ball!"

Moments earlier, I had been hanging upside down like a bat, thighs gripping a metal pole, wondering if the pole fitness class I had signed up for was really what I wanted to be doing.

Physically, I was in the best shape of my life—long gone were the extra pounds and rounded shape I earned during my recent pregnancy as I spent more and more days every week exercising to my maximum. Being so fit made me feel invincible, bursting with energy and vibrating with endorphins, secretly reveling in the admiring looks of my gym buddies and other friends.

Then I crashed.

My teacher, who was supposed to be spotting me in a move definitely not designed for beginners, let go of me as I fell headfirst eighteen inches to the ground. There were no mats underneath the pole.

> *"I remember the strange calmness I felt, lying on the floor, aware of being conscious yet dazed."*

I remember the strange calmness I felt, lying on the floor, aware of being conscious yet dazed. In a weird moment of synchronicity, the fire alarm in the fitness studio began ringing as I fell and continued ringing as I left to go to the hospital.

The interns who examined me looked at my jammed neck and declared that I was fine. I knew what day it was and how to count by nines; I guess these are things you might forget if you've had a concussion. I left the hospital thinking a few days' rest and ice for my neck would set me right and I'd be back to the gym, though maybe not to the pole, once again.

It turned out I still had a lot of healing—and learning—yet to do.

Will I ever fully recover? Will my life be this way forever? These were the questions that circled around and around inside my head for months, demanding a response. Unfortunately, I had none.

The term "recovery" is a loaded one for concussion survivors. We count the months since the event with the attentiveness of a prisoner marking time on the walls of their cell; we look to survivors further along their healing paths with anxious, hopeful eyes, pleading with them to tell us they're fully recovered and what their magic cure was. We live in dread that we will not recover the parts of ourselves that were lost when we were injured. We crave certainty when nothing in life is truly certain.

There will come a day perhaps when we lose count of the months passing, when we stop comparing ourselves to others. Maybe we will begin to feel a subtle shift in our attitude towards our injury that doesn't focus exclusively on "full recovery" but instead on "healing." Like life, healing is a journey rather than a destination, a process rather than a result.

Maybe we can slowly begin to back away from that big hole at the center of our lives, the concussion that has taken so much away from us and has become our chronic preoccupation: resenting it, fearing it, identifying with it. We can allow the good things in our lives to continue to have importance and not get swallowed up by the pain we feel.

Does switching out of "full recovery" thinking mean we are giving up on ever being recovered? No. Accepting that we are on a healing journey with others who can help will remove pressure from the brain, which creates the most favorable conditions for recovery.

What do we do in-between appointments with members of our health team, those skilled healers who bring relief for our painful symptoms and reassurance for our troubled minds? I know I often leaned heavily on them, gobbling up every word and piece of advice, desperate for good news about my condition. I also wanted to experience the same feeling of knowledgeable comfort outside of office visits, when doubts crept in.

I explored the idea of being my own therapist, of re-imagining the pleasurable or meaningful activities of my daily living as actually therapeutic. An hour in the garden, a walk around the neighborhood, peeling carrots for supper—I visualized each task as just as important to my healing as ninety minutes with a physiotherapist, doing dizzying balance exercises.

A learned skill, self-healing is one that can transform our lives, even if we are not injured. It removes the pressure of deadlines and accommodates the slower pace the brain needs to heal. When we are not in a rush, we notice amazing things and make true progress in our learning and healing.

The movement practice of NIA (short for neuro-integrative muscular activity) introduced me to the concept of self-healing through acts of kindness to the self and especially to the body, which may be feeling left out with all the attention typically given to the brain after a concussion. In the NIA philosophy, "Learning to perform acts of self-kindness comes from tracking 'feel good' sensations. When you foster self-healing through acts of kindness you naturally become more proactive and in control of outcomes. You replace the attitude of, 'My shoulder is hurting,' to one of, 'I am healing my shoulder.'" *(Debbie Rosas, co-founder of NIA)*

This shift in how we speak and think about our injury and its effect on our lives does not deny the presence of pain and sadness, but it can help to empower us when we feel powerless. During my healing, I reframed my most persistent complaint from "I'm having a bad day with lots of concussion symptoms," to "This is a good day to focus on self-healing." I also began to redefine my relationship with fear when I changed "I am feeling anxiety," to "I'm learning to be a calm person."

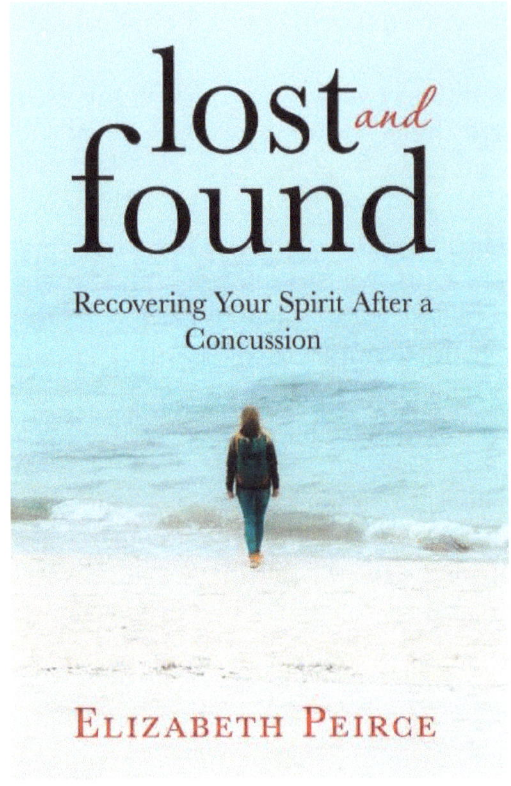

This language shift helped me see my task as part of a process, one that might take a long time. Giving myself permission to contemplate a longer recovery time relieved the pressure I had been putting on myself to heal quickly. It was a great gift.

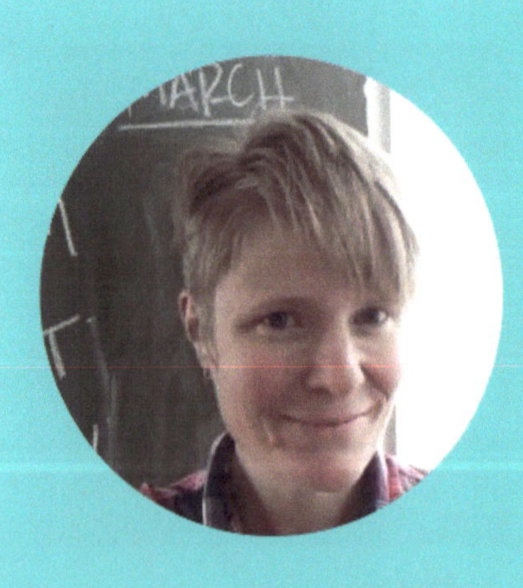

Meet Elizabeth Peirce

Elizabeth Peirce is an author, editor and teacher living in Halifax, Nova Scotia. Her latest book Lost and Found: Recovering Your Spirit After A Concussion, *is based on her own TBI experience and is an empowering toolkit of strategies designed to activate the innate healing potential of the concussion survivor. Learn more at elizabethpeirce.ca.*

CONCUSSIONS & SPORTS

Concussions are brain injuries and are ravaging the nation, from little leagues to professionals. As the parent of a child involved in sports, it is critical that you recognize the signs of concussion and seek medical assistance immediately.

The Facts About Concussion In Sports

300,000 the number of sports related concussions in the USA each year.

1,215 concussions were diagnosed in the NFL between 2012 and 2016.

25% of concussion sufferers fail to get assessed by medical personel.

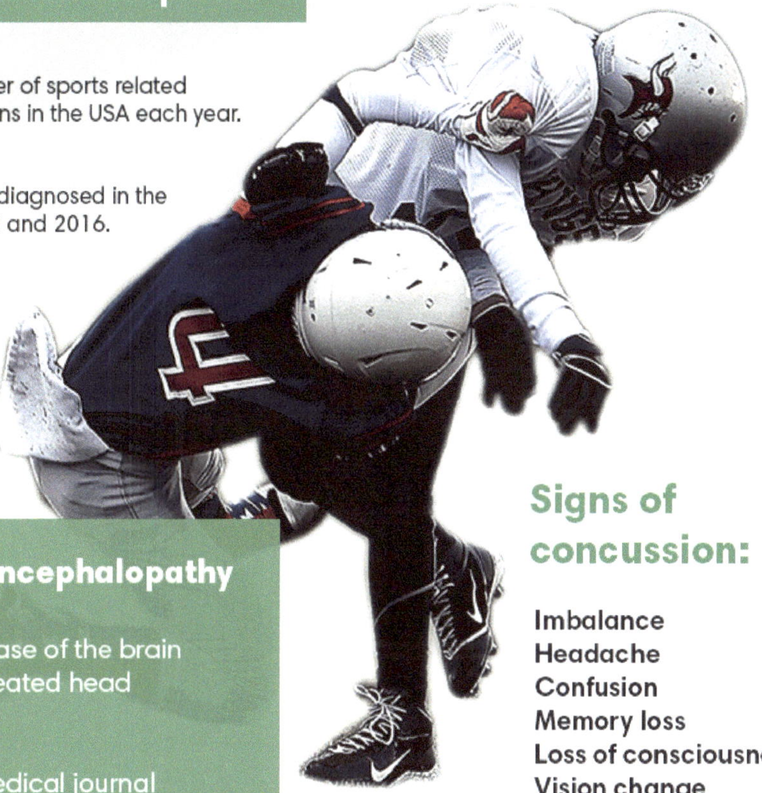

Chronic Traumatic Encephalopathy

CTE is a degenerative disease of the brain and is associated with repeated head traumas like concussions.

A study published in the medical journal JAMA identified CTE in 99% of deceased NFL players' brains that were donated to scientific research.

Signs of concussion:

Imbalance
Headache
Confusion
Memory loss
Loss of consciousness
Vision change
Hearing change
Mood change
Fatigue
Malaise

Call your doctor if you answer yes to any of the following:

1. Is my child acting abnormally?
2. Does my child seem more drowsy than normal?
3. Has his or her behavior changed?

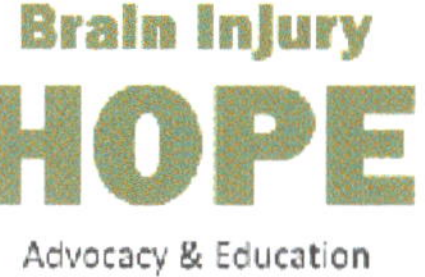

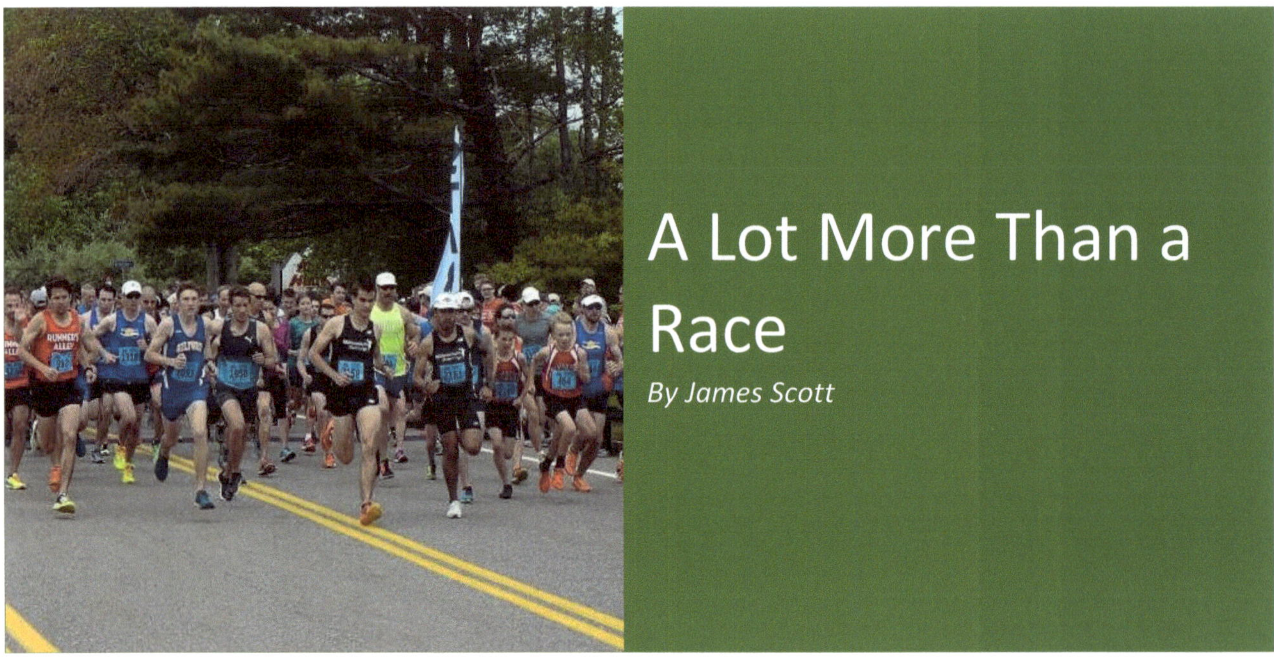

A Lot More Than a Race

By James Scott

I certainly haven't counted them all, but based on the numerous t-shirts I see, there must be thoudsands of road race participants every year. So why, you ask, am I highlighting one of them? Well, as many of these races are memorials and/or fundraisers for worthy causes, one in particular, the Runner's Alley Redhook Memorial 5k is one with which I have a very personal connection.

Portsmouth, NH's Krempels Center (KC) benefits from 100% of the proceeds of this annual race which completed its 21st edition on Memorial Day weekend of 2018. While the course is great for fast running and many impressive times are earned each year, I have to believe that's only a small part of this community favorite's appeal. Many area businesses attend and offer samples of their products. The post-race festivities become more of a party resembling a large family's reunion. Race participants also receive a sample of one of Redhook's fine brews in a commemorative glass. The day's festivities kick off

> *"Being a KC member also means that I am a brain injury survivor, serving those living with acquired brain injury from trauma, tumor, or stroke."*

with a kids' fun run. While I don't have any kids of my own, I hope to see my godson out there soon.

There is an incredible amount of fun had by all who participate each spring. There is also tremendous financial support for Krempels Center generated by the race. What makes my experience with the Runner's Alley Redhook Memorial 5k so relevant? Well… being a member of Krempels Center means a lot of things. I benefit greatly from the tireless work by an organization carrying out David Krempels vision (he is a TBI survivor himself and the KC founder) and KC's beautiful mission of "improving the lives of people living with brain injury."

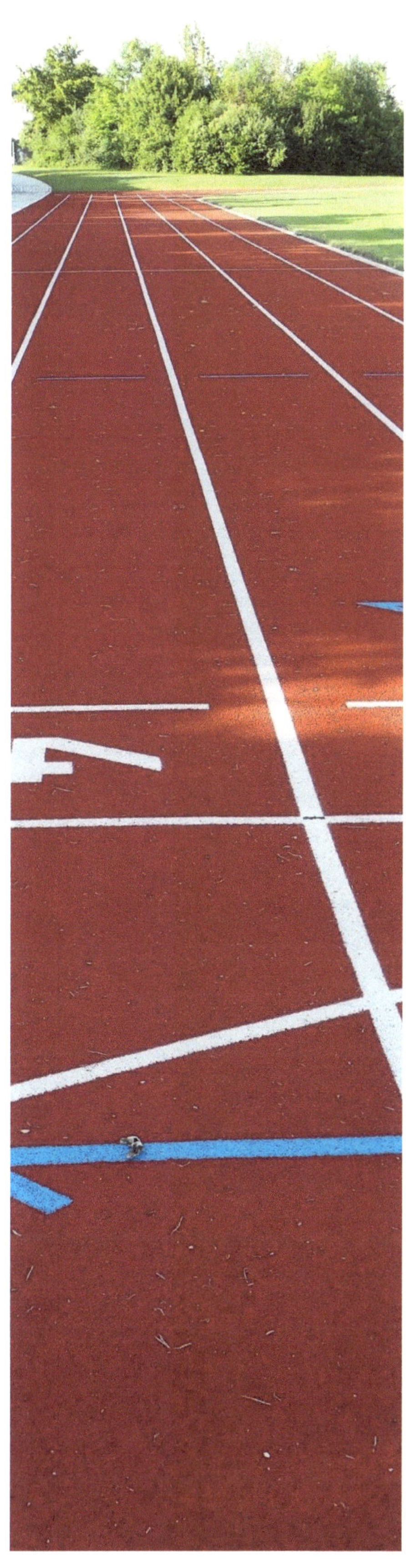

Being a KC member also means that I am a brain injury survivor, serving those living with acquired brain injury from trauma, tumor, or stroke. KC runs a community-based model rather than the traditional medical services facility. In fact, I like to think of the incredibly valuable rehab services like physical, occupational, and speech therapy as where you learn how to function, while KC provides a supportive community where you can begin to actually live a new life.

The Runner's Alley Redhook Memorial 5k is one of KC's main fundraising events with KC benefiting from the days' proceeds. As part of the Seacoast Race Series, it is one of eight annual races that are supported by the enthusiastic running community of the Seacoast NH area. The Series is a really cool synergy of people combining self-improvement with events benefiting great non-profits improving the community.

Fundraising is vital to Krempels' operation. Although anyone, anytime can acquire a brain injury in one of the many ways in which this devastating injury can occur, Acquired Brain Injury (ABI) is not one of the well-known conditions in the forefront of people's minds. Neither my immediate or extended family had any awareness of the Krempels Center prior to the early stages of my recovery. It truly is amazing that such a beautiful organization dedicated to improving the lives of acquired brain injury survivors is such a hidden gem. Although, with so many worthy causes, tragedies, and natural disasters in the twenty-four hour news cycle, I shouldn't be too surprised.

While I could go on and on expressing my gratitude for David Krempels' generosity to survivors in establishing the organization now supported by private donations and fundraisers, I'd really like to explain why this topic intrigued me. While it's not much of a leap to connect running for self-improvement to a road race fundraising for a non-profit dedicated to improving lives, it's the similarity between running and brain injury recovery that I find amazing. Let me start off by telling you a bit about my own involvement in running.

One look and you can see that I don't have the prototypical runner's body, tall and lanky; rather the exact opposite, short and stocky. In fact, I would describe my relationship with running prior to acquiring a TBI *(Traumatic Brain Injury)* July 4th, 2006, as "I guess, if I have to." I only ran when required to by an athletic coach or at the gym. I know that this is hardly inspiring, however, I really believe running has been vital to my physical recovery.

Recovering from a brain injury is something that you never actually finish. At times, my progress seems to happen in leaps and bounds, while at other times the pace seems glacial. Brain injury recovery has a lot in common with many other types of self-improvement, particularly running. I'm the first to admit how incredibly fortunate that I've been in my recovery in all areas of my recovery- physical, cognitive rehabilitation, social, support networks (both family and otherwise), and perhaps mostly for being a KC member. Even with all these factors helping, life isn't always perfect, and doing the daily work to improve my ability to participate in life becomes daunting at times.

Sometimes I wake up and my muscles are especially tight, with a clenched left hand making tying my shoes impossible, or despite having slept a full night, awaken in nothing short of an exhausted state. On these days I think to myself, "You've got to be kidding me. All these years of hard work and I'm not done struggling yet." While not quite the exact same sentiment, I often find myself sulking and having a one-person pity party over having to lace up my sneakers for what feels like the millionth day in a row to get a workout in. It would be a lie for me to say I leap out of bed rearing to go for a run and never feel that all the previous jogs should make me automatically fit and athletic.

So what keeps me going? While it isn't one specific thing, or certainly public adulation coupled with fame and fortune resulting from my running speed, I can identify one powerful motivator: Every year at the Runner's Alley Redhook I've managed to set a new personal best 5k time! While not breaking the tape at the finish line, or even finishing in the top half for that matter, each year's finish serves as confirmation that I'm doing something right.

I wish I could say that my perspective on life is always great now or that I never find myself overcome with self-pity, but I'm only human. As, Ted, a fellow KC member who I've become close with over the years, replies when I inquire "How are you?" "A little better each day," says Ted. I guess if I can take the liberty of amending Ted's response to, "A little faster each Runner's Alley Redhook Memorial 5k," this statement means that I'm moving in the right direction!

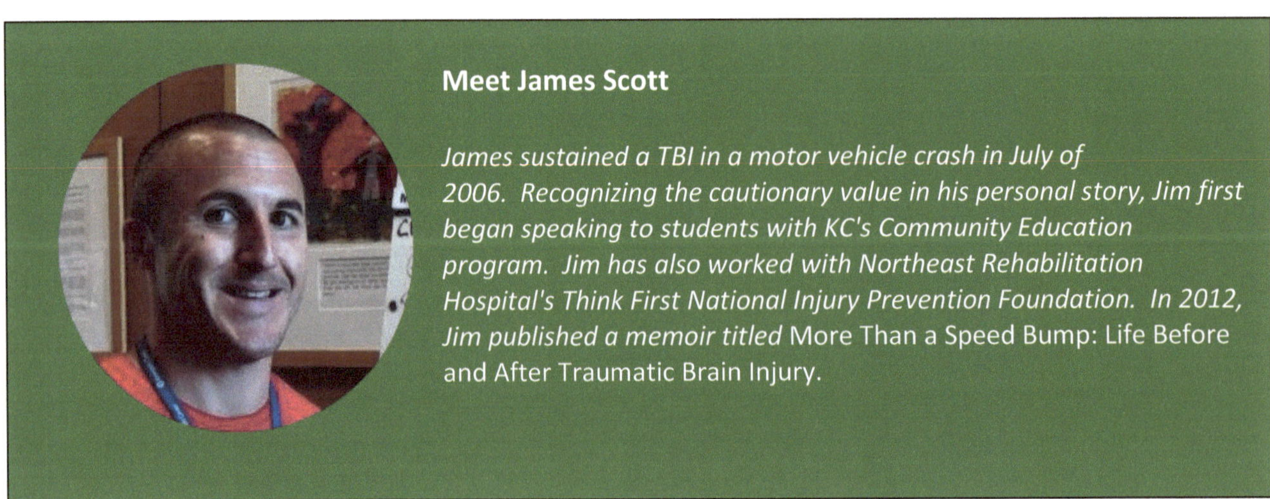

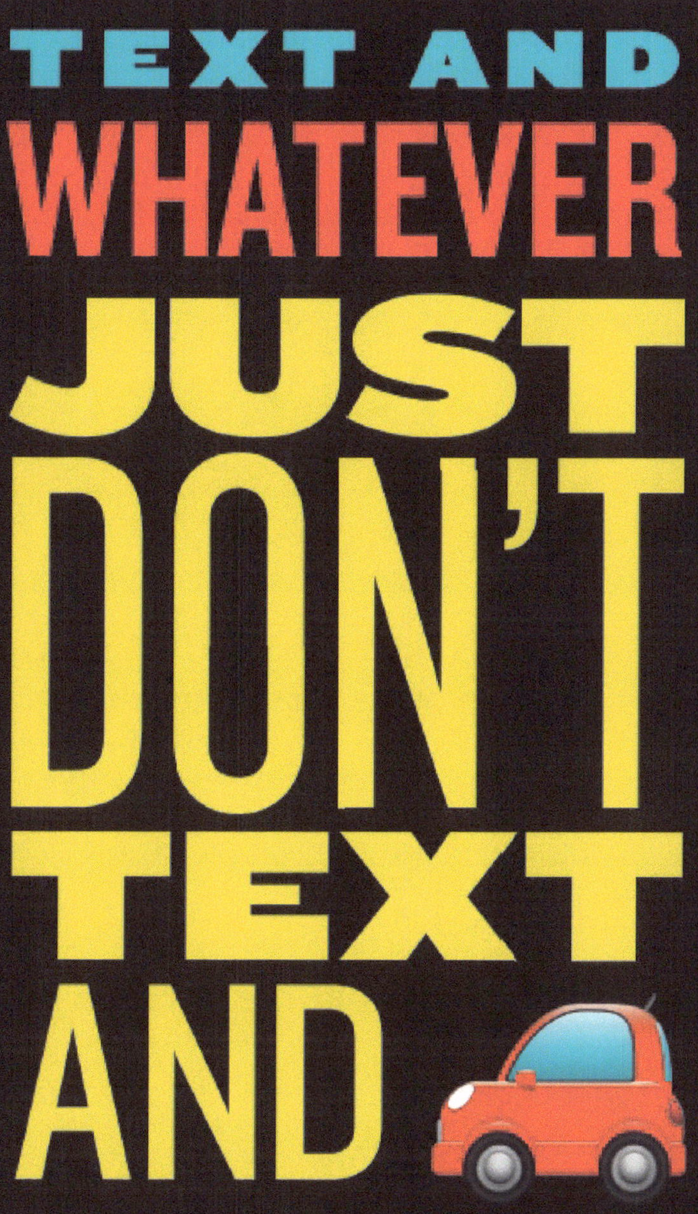

TEXT AND
WHATEVER
JUST
DON'T
TEXT
AND
STOPTEXTSSTOPWRECKS.ORG

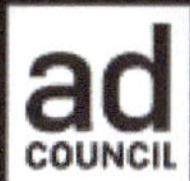

ad
COUNCIL
NHTSA

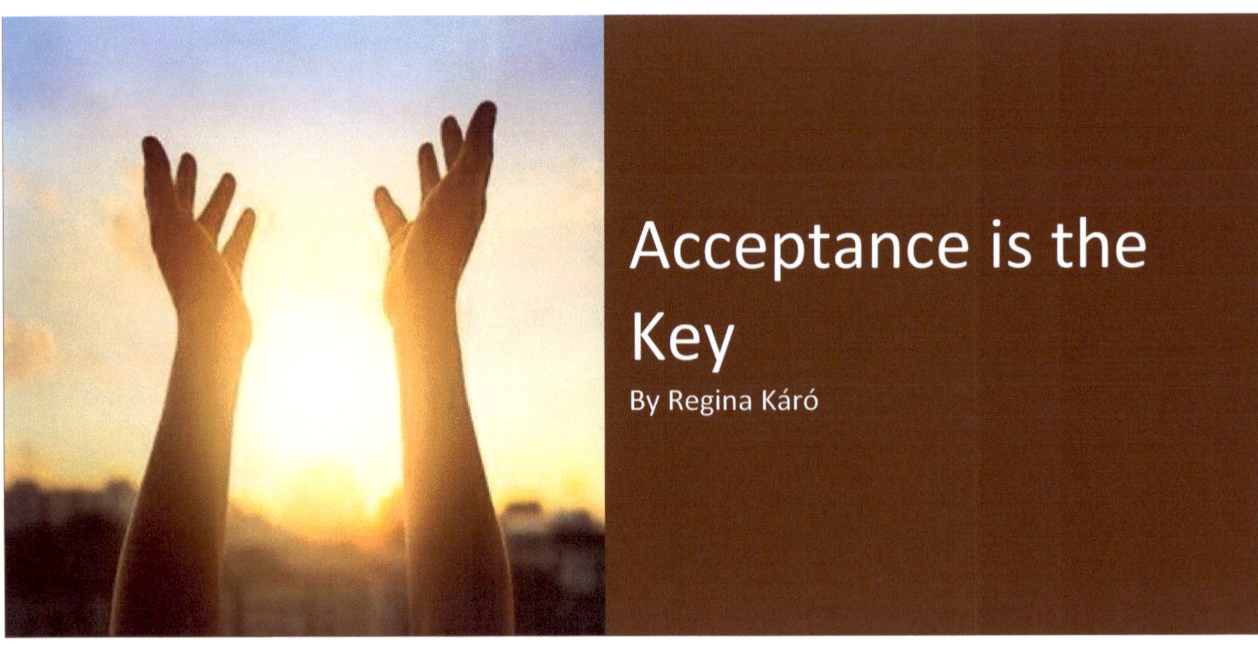

I was a big dreamer, a Hungarian girl trying to prove her best in an American hotel as a server. One night I was cycling home from work and got hit by a car. The lights of the car weren't turned on, or the guy who was driving was on his phone, or perhaps I wasn't paying enough attention. We'll never know, and I don't think it would be easier if I knew. The accident happened and this trip home nearly took my life.

I was in coma for months, and a vegetative state afterwards. I slowly regained consciousness. I had to learn a lot of things again and attempt to restart my life. I returned home and started thinking about my future. I wanted my life back to where I was a good server and living an active life. I was the life and soul of the party many times. I wanted that back and I wanted to continue just where I left off. Needless to say, that would be impossible and crazy.

> *"I was in coma for months and a vegetative state afterwards. I slowly regained consciousness. I had to learn a lot of things again and attempt to restart my life."*

At first, I thought that it would only take time. A little time and everything would be the same. I started again the relationship I had before. I left out of consideration that I already ended that relationship. I had friends I thought would stay next to me no matter what happened. I thought I could rebuild old friendships. "Maybe this time it's gonna be different," and "Everybody deserves a second chance."

Nobody proved that either of my beliefs were right. Second chances were like giving them another chance to lead me on. An accident like this is a test for every relationship. At least now I know who my true friends are. At the same time, I didn't want the personality I used to have back. I was happy with many things that had changed. Dual feelings experiencing a change in life are part of the grieving process.

Eventually I realized that I had to get used to everything as it was now and try to benefit from what had happened to me. I joined a personality development program. There the girl told us to try to ask ourselves a few questions.

I asked myself, "What if I don't HAVE to be the same?" Meaning I don't have to react the way I used to. I don't have to wear the clothes with the same style. I don't have to think the same. I CAN try new things. Only if I weren't so afraid to be different. I was different enough because of the visible results of my injury. I wanted to get lost in the crowd. I just wanted to be normal again!

It was a long time until I understood that being different or standing out from the crowd is only being ME. There isn't a problem with not knowing what the next step is, like I always did. There isn't a problem with restarting my life. It isn't a problem that I have to learn new things. It's difficult, sure it is. But there are other people starting to learn a new profession. If they can learn, why can't I?

Getting out of my comfort zone can be challenging but it's necessary. Allowing myself to feel how I feel is important. I knew how and what should I feel in certain situations. I needed to accept that I feel different things now. Not in a supernatural way, but things have changed in my head.

I had to be strong. Instead of holding on to the past, it was necessary to let go of my ingrained habits and thoughts. I always wanted to do the right thing, but what if there is no ultimate right? What I think is right may be totally wrong from another perspective. Still I wanted to be perfectly normal like anybody else.

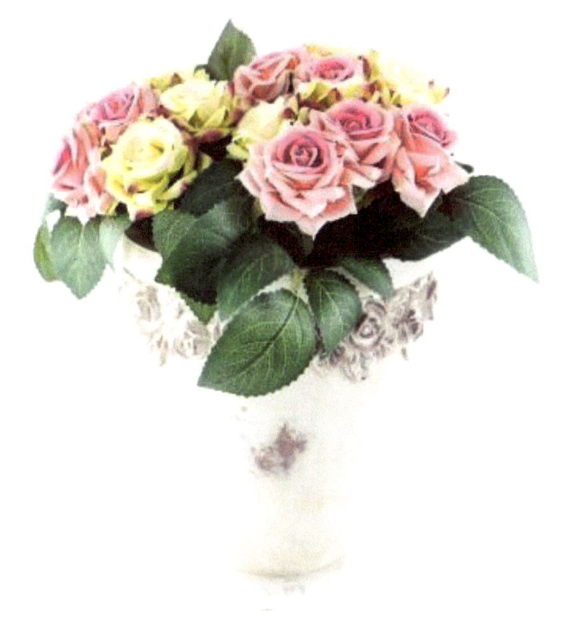

But what's the use in that? Who decides what normal looks like? Who would really benefit from that? If I try to be somebody else, I never can be true to myself. I had to be brave and start exploring this new version of me. It's exciting. It's freedom to know that I can be anything. I needed and still need to eliminate limiting people and limiting beliefs from my life.

After all I can say that life is truly wonderful. Being different, not being able to speak like I used to, not being able to walk or use my right hand like before are challenging, but every day something new happens, something different than before. Sometimes it's hard to find the positive, but it's worth the search.

I've also learned things in the hospital, I've become a different person. I've learned that only good things take us forward, and that patience and respect are important. I've experienced that being in a vulnerable situation is one of the hardest things in the world and I've learned that in our hearts and souls there has to be peace. We have to accept the unchangeable things. Once we accepted the things we cannot change, we can start healing.

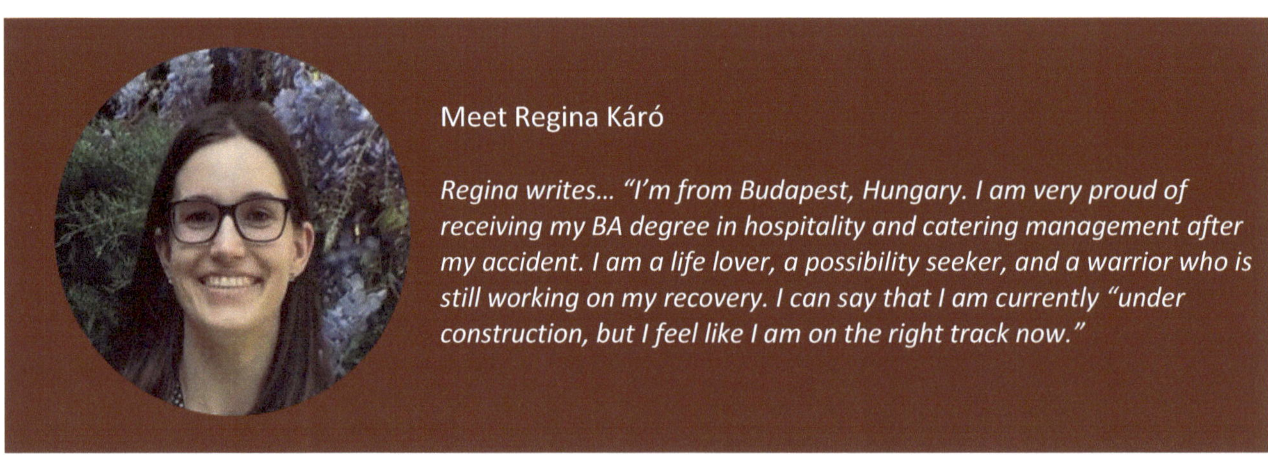

Meet Regina Káró

Regina writes… "I'm from Budapest, Hungary. I am very proud of receiving my BA degree in hospitality and catering management after my accident. I am a life lover, a possibility seeker, and a warrior who is still working on my recovery. I can say that I am currently "under construction, but I feel like I am on the right track now."

Join our Facebook Family

What do almost 30,000 people from 60 countries and five continents all have in common? They are all members of our vibrant Facebook family at /TBIHopeandInspiration

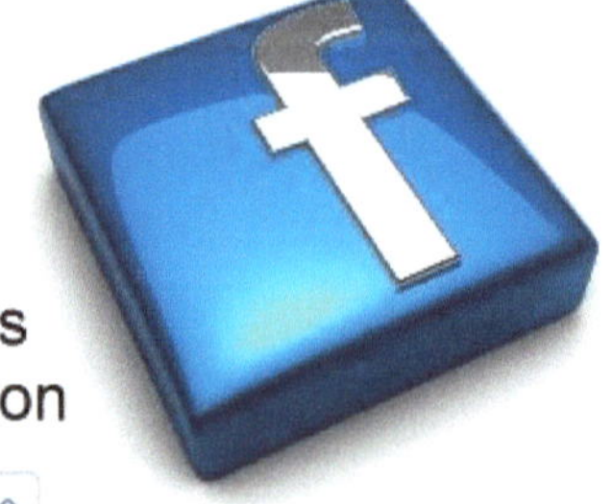

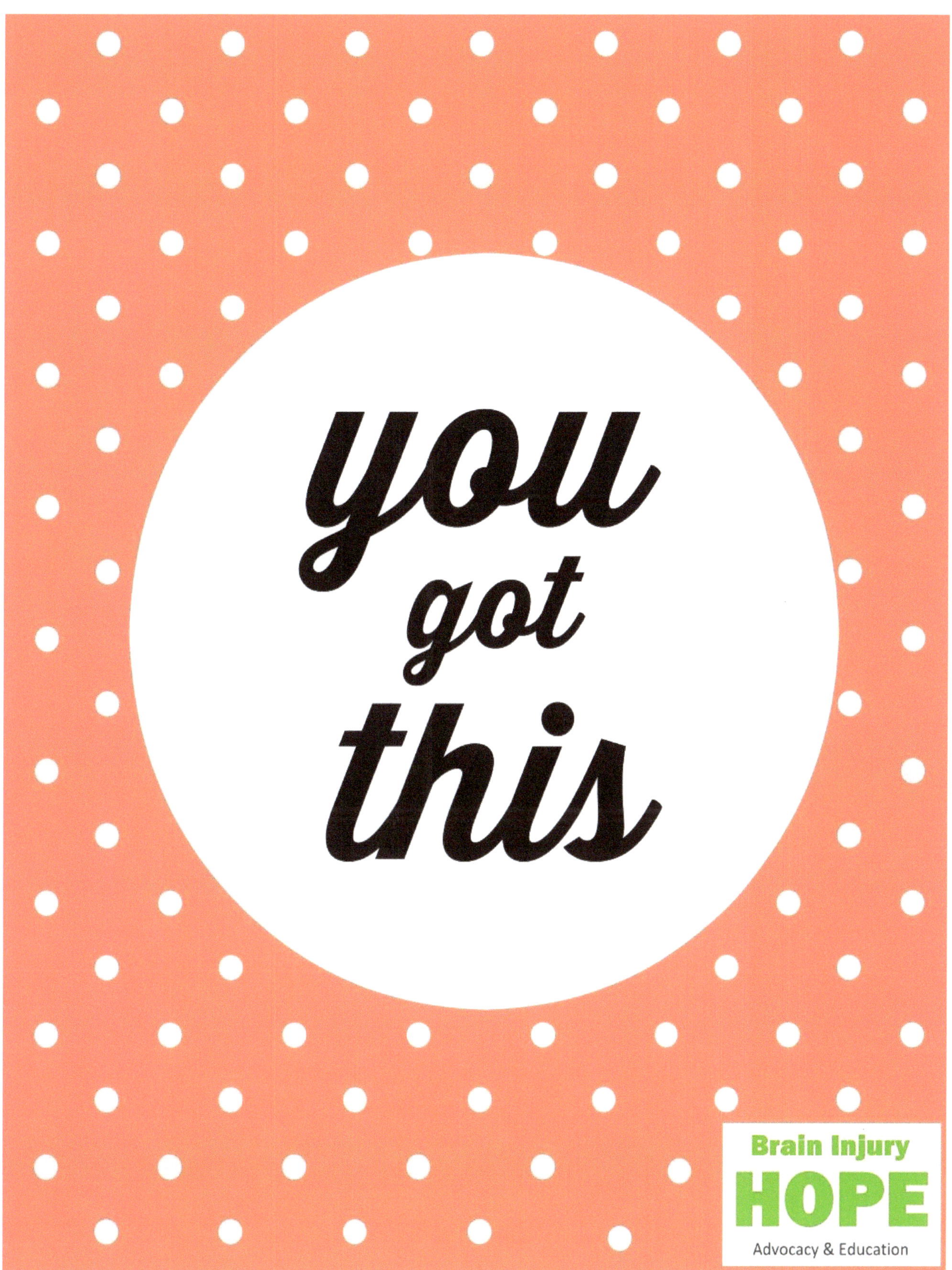

you
got
this

Brain Injury
HOPE
Advocacy & Education

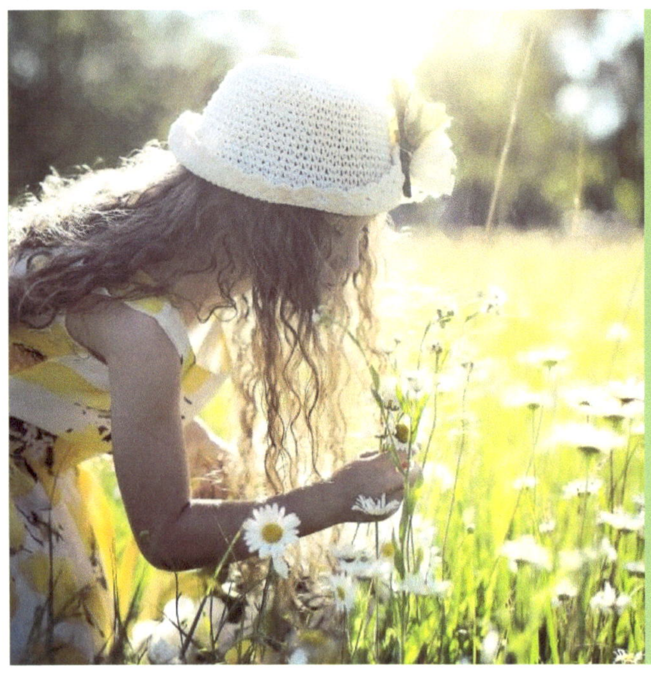

I Choose Joy

By Andrea Rauser

Over a year-and-a-half into my recovery from a *'mild closed head injury,'* every morning provides a difficult decision for me to make. Before I open my eyes, I wonder if this will be my first symptom free day. Then I do a head check and open my eyes realizing that no, it's not today. I had a concussion when I was a toddler and whiplash in the nineteen-eighties. I then suffered another concussion two years prior to this one. Fortunately, those symptoms cleared in less than two weeks.

Life was great and we were all healthy and well. We had just celebrated a beautiful family Christmas vacation time together, and both of my girls were back in school. In the blink of an eye everything changed. I was doing dishes and glanced in the next room where my favorite coffee cup was teasing me to be washed too. While the water was running, I foolishly decided to dash and get it. All I dashed into was an open cupboard door to the top of my head. I scrambled and my life was flipped upside down instantly.

> *"The beginning was by far one of the most difficult journeys I've ever had, and there have already been way too many for this middle-aged body."*

The beginning was by far one of the most difficult journeys I've ever had, and there have already been way too many for this middle-aged body. I went back to college and switched careers in 2010, becoming an Education Assistant with high school and grade school special needs students. I thank this path of my life for giving me the knowledge and skill to be able to accommodate my symptoms with tricks and compassion without any personal concerns of vanity.

I was lucky as the vestibular portion of my concussion turned around almost quickly with a physiotherapist and osteopath working in a concussion center in my city. Unfortunately, I have had a moderate to severe headache and varied amounts of brain fog every day since.

I now get to wear two pairs of glasses, instead of my super convenient Progressive lenses, but the vision therapy and prisms are working somewhat.

I can actually drive my car again on roads I know well and am comfortable on. What Joy! Screens are still limited and TV as well. Audiobooks are amazing and I have read so much. Word Search books are great for keeping the language part of my brain working. What joy! Sleep… where to even begin, not enough, too much, can't sleep, can't wake up, it's a flip of the coin. I am so thankful for audiobooks and guided meditations that can help me on the restless nights to get to the point of relaxation that my body requires now. I love that when I wake up, even though every symptom is still there, they have decreased slightly, and I know that my body is healing.

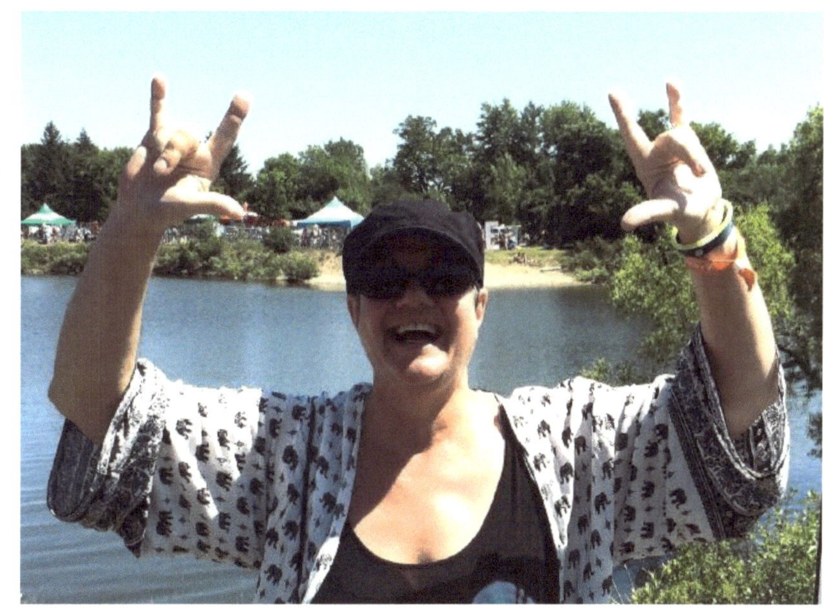

The tinnitus is that bonus gift with concussion that no one really mentions. You don't understand until it starts and does not stop. I found a great app that works sometimes, but the best way is to ignore it, and give it no attention at all. Sometimes you can actually forget that it is annoying.

Worse for me is the audio input overstimulation. Magically I found musicians earplugs work great and are super easy to pop in and out. I always have them on me. I get a bit stubborn and will wait until everything is too loud and my head is spinning, then in they go. I close my eyes and take a mini break. What joy!

Not being able to understand verbal or written instructions easily is annoying, and conversations coming to a complete halt because of my beautiful brain are as well. Thankfully, all my family and close friends really get this, and we laugh when it happens, instead of being super frustrated. What joy!

The memory loss symptom is a real bummer sometimes, but then again, I'm always learning new things. My startle and fight or flight response is set very high now. When it happens, the others around me are usually just as surprised and startled by my reaction to the stimuli, which makes us laugh. Dressed in all my armor which includes my hat, glasses and earplugs, when I venture out into the world, I always let salesclerks or anyone I start a conversation with know that I am in concussion recovery and may exhibit symptoms. When I suddenly stop talking, say the wrong word or close my eyes, there is no confusion and I find this disclosure makes every interaction go better.

We have spent so much money on well over a dozen different therapies hoping for the golden bullet that will fix me, but unfortunately there doesn't seem to be any. I have tried energy work with many different practitioners who all have helped me find the peace and joy during this difficult time.

Instead of being completely engulfed in how much grief I feel about being unemployable with no long term benefits and no money, I look around at what I do have. I have a beautiful home, loving family and great friends. Grieving who I was and who I thought I was going to be bursts out of me numerous times a day, but I am honoring that this is who I am for now and that's absolutely okay.

I'm not giving up, and I am still going to continue looking for my golden bullet. I accept that the Universe has slowed my forward journey and that's okay too. So every morning when I wake up, one of the first things I say to myself is, "I choose JOY." I am not saying that this is easy, but for me it is so much healthier to try to find any glimmer of hope and run with it, rather than wallow in all that has changed my life. Today I choose JOY!

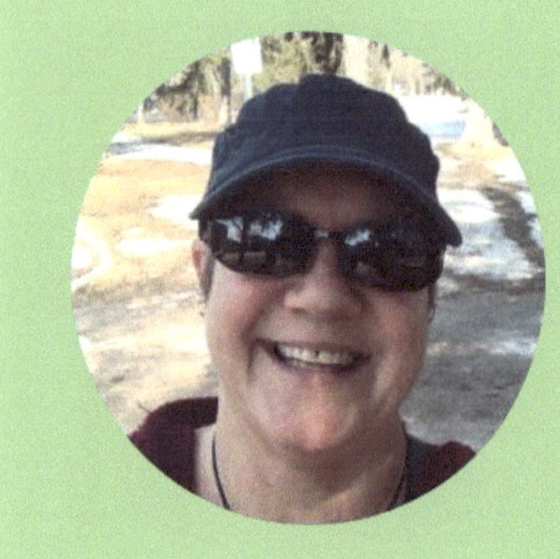

Meet Andrea Rauser

Andrea writes… "I am 56 years old, and live in my hometown of Guelph, Ontario with my husband Erick who is a manufacturing teacher. I have two daughters in University who are both home for the summer, so it's been super loud and filled with joy. I am fortunate to have my sister living nearby and she has been very generous with her time helping me get around, as well as helping me to understand what information I may have been given. I am so happy my mother lives close and our daily communication helps keep me grounded."

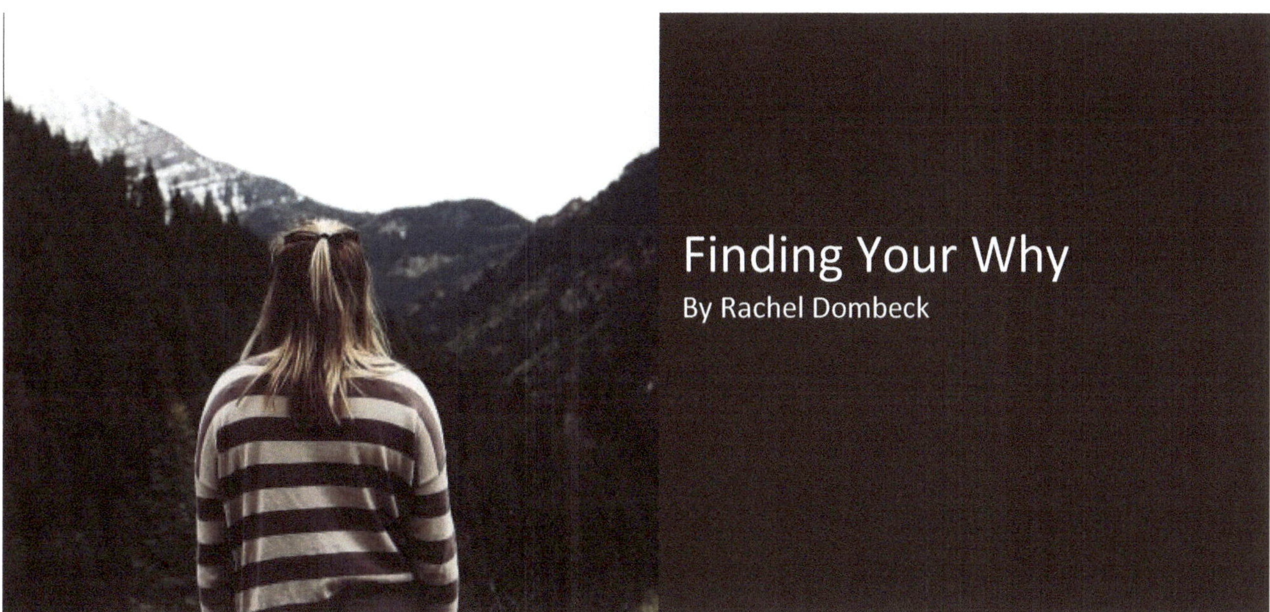

The things I am about to talk about are not easy, not fun, but they are real and need to be brought up. They need to be talked about in love and kindness, in truth and hope, because, isn't that why we are all here? To find some glimmer, glimpse, faint sight of hope?

Let me be frank. You need to have a Why right now in your life. You HAVE to have a why. You require one. Your WHY is what will get you up in the morning in the pain, headaches, migraines, brain fog, extreme fatigue. Your WHY is what will keep you going from one moment to the next when you literally don't know how you are going to do one more moment like this, let alone days, weeks, months, and even years.

"The rate of suicide of individuals with any kind of brain injury is horribly high and tragically happens all too often."

Having a WHY in front of you keeps you going through the worst days and moments, the good and bad doctors' appointments, the good news and the disappointing news. If you do not have a WHY for why you won't give up, well then you just might give up.

I had nights, more than I care to admit, where I would pray to not wake up. I would say, "I am tired of pain, of feeling like I'm failing, of feeling useless, and I just don't want to take up space here and have no point so just let me be done with this already! If there is still a point, and still something - still hope, then I'll wake up in my bed in the morning." I woke up, in my bed, in my room, in my mom's house, and thought, "Alright, let's do this another day." Weary, tired, in pain, and still without any more answers than the night before, I would pull myself out of bed to face yet another day.

The rate of suicide of individuals with any kind of brain injury is horribly high and tragically happens all too often. I don't have statistics for you because honestly, I don't think I need a number to throw out at you. If you are reading this, you know because you either know someone who has struggled with it or you have thought about it yourself.

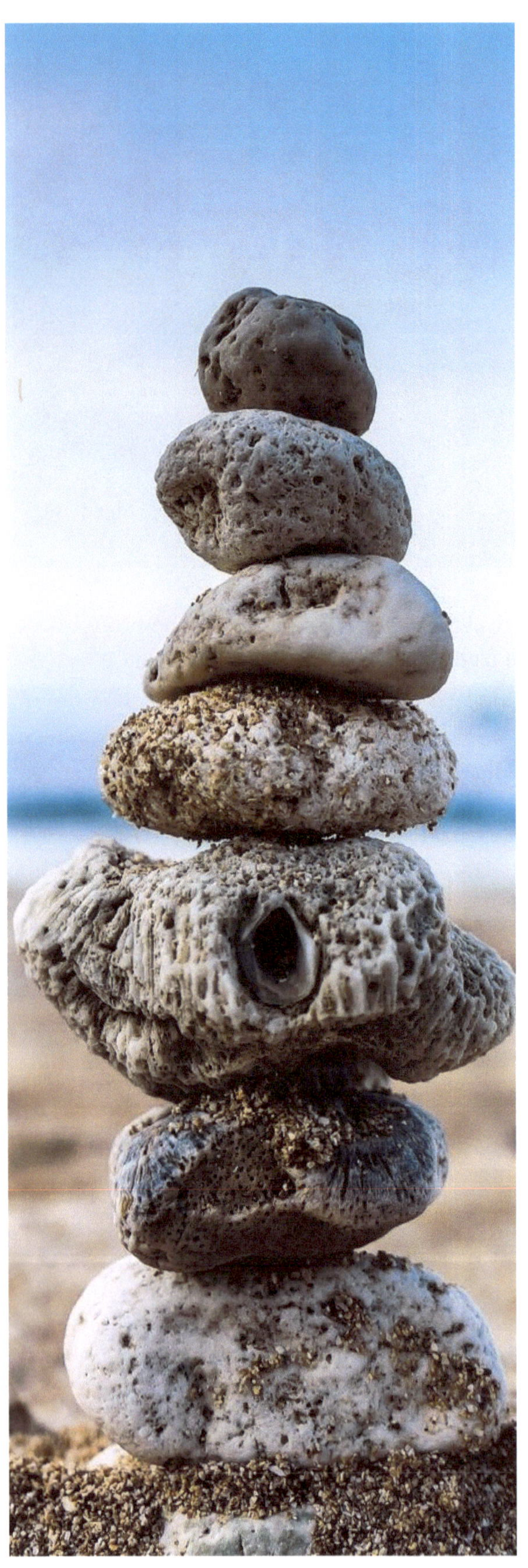

I am fighting back the tears the whole time I am writing this part of my story because I remember the darkest, deepest, blackest moments up till now, and I do not want anyone to have to face those times and not come through them, to keep sinking deeper when there IS HOPE and there IS LIGHT and there IS LIFE to be lived even after a TBI. BUT the truth is I can't help you, others can't, unless you help yourself.

In the dark painful moments, whether it's the pressure of the physical pain, the loss of friends, job, home, health, the loneliness in recovery, a let down from the latest doctor's report, another financial blow, whatever the trigger is this time, the dark moments are scary. The best way I can describe it is feeling out of control, breathless, suffocating, paralyzed, emotionally imploding. Oh, I would want to scream and punch and hit things, and wish I had superpowers like Wonder Woman so I could just put my arms together and blow everything up. I may have even tried. What do you do when you're crying so hard you almost choke, and it hurts so much you think you might just pass out from the pain, when you curl up in the corner and cover yourself in a blanket but know you can't live that way? How do you do this?

I took one tiny step at a time, and I want to share that with you in hopes that it might save a life, or at least offer a faint glimmer of light in your bleakest, darkest moment to know you are not alone, you are not worthless, or a failure. There is hope and absolutely, positively most of all know that you are stronger than you will ever know.

Find your WHY. It doesn't have to be grand or earth-changing or anything, it is your why and no one else's so it can literally be anything; but find it, know it. My main WHY is my nieces and nephews. I want them to know they can face anything, be anything and they can do anything they put their mind to. But if I quit, if I give up, what does that tell them? What will they have to live with then? I learned to picture each of their faces very vividly so when my dark depression and loneliness hit, when pain seemed suffocating, I would visualize my WHY to keep sticking it out, to keep going through this seemingly endless tunnel of

TBI recovery and keep putting one foot in front of the other. Since we are already getting nitty gritty real here, I will tell you I would also visualize them if I did give up, if I did take the easy way out of life.

Learn the difference between *fact* and *feeling*. Yours, mine--our feelings are real and we need to acknowledge them and face them, but we must know and remember that they are not necessarily facts. I can feel like a failure; that doesn't mean I am one. I can feel like there is no hope; that doesn't mean there isn't. I can feel like I don't know how to face another day; that doesn't mean there aren't answers there. We must not let our feelings consume us into a black hole of despair and worthlessness.

Breathe. Just. Breathe. Sometimes, you just need to sit and take a deep breath in, and out. And do it again. And again. And again. And again. It is one of the simplest, most overlooked and underused techniques to get through a panic or anxiety attack.

Go to bed - literally. Sometimes we just need to rest--our minds, our brains, and our bodies. TBI can be fatiguing in ways I didn't think were possible, so sometimes now I just tell myself, "Girl, you're tired. Let's go to bed and face this with a rested brain tomorrow." Yes, I talk to myself like that. And yes, it helps a lot. Reach out. Reach out to someone. Even if just to tell them, "Hey, I'm not good right now. I'm in a dark place. I just don't think I can do this." Sometimes we just need to feel heard, seen, acknowledged. Have an outside viewpoint from someone who can see us better than we can see ourselves and our life in that moment.

Look beyond the immediate and beyond yourself. It is vital to remember that the reason we feel like things are hopeless or useless, or we are considering an out to this life, is because we are not able to conceive things being any other way for the foreseeable future.

"Have an outside viewpoint from someone who can see us better than we can see ourselves and our life in that moment."

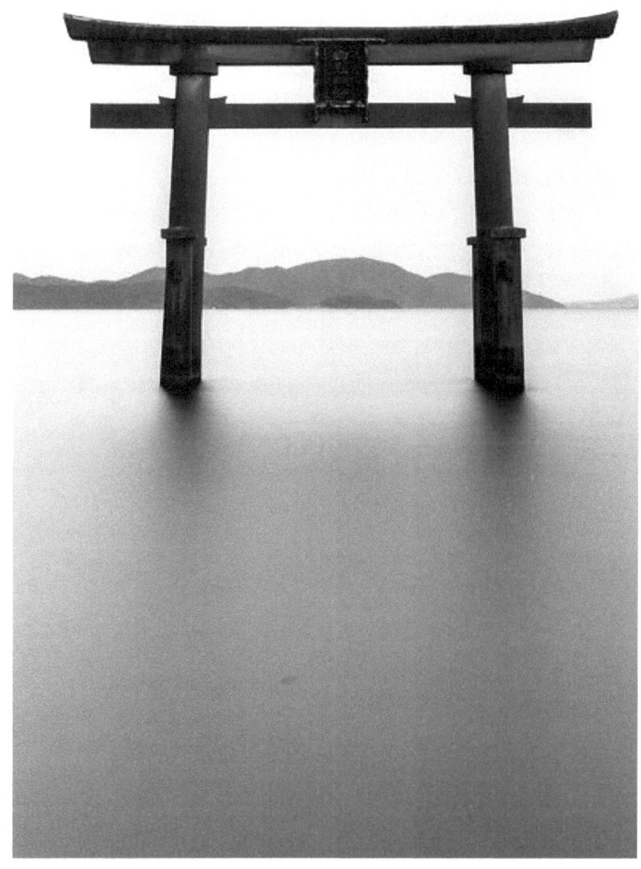

When that bleakest, colorless, void future is what we see in that moment, it destroys our will to continue, if we let it--if we dwell on it and let ourselves stay in that and wallow, which is why this then circles back around to having a WHY. When you are in that moment, you are in a battle and the weapon that you must use to fight back the darkness with is your WHY.

The picture of my nieces and nephews in my mind has brought me out of the darkest moments and given me the courage to face another day, even if I have no more answers than I did before, and even if the pain is still there and just as intense. My healing and recovery moved forward exponentially (and still does) when I shifted my focus outward to someone else. It doesn't have to be anything huge. It can be texting a friend to say hello, thinking of you, sending you hugs even if I can't physically go out and hang out with friends. It can be sending a card to someone. Whatever you have to do, just reach out. When we are in a dark hole of our own, it's easy to think we are the only ones. We have it the worst; no one else is there too. It's dark, so we can't see them. But the truth is we are actually all so much more alike than we are different.

It is challenging to explain the dark places a TBI can take you on any given day. It can be with or without warning...maybe because you overdid it, or maybe because you did everything right, and you still ended up in a Post-Concussion Symptom black hole. When you find yourself in one of those, you know the battle to get out is not so much about "fighting through," but "flowing through," taking one step at a time.

It is very easy and common with TBI to have emotions all over the place, be irrational, up and down, and have a challenged perspective of the reality of the situation. It is easy to feel like things are hopeless and bleak. You become susceptible to feeling depressed, anxious and overwhelmed in a matter of seconds. Fellow TBI warriors understand this. We don't like it. We hate it, rather. But I'm sure you're reading this and nodding your head in agreement and can relate all too well.

What does all of this have to do with knowing your WHY? Your WHY is going to be a huge part of you getting out of that place. When you are in the blackest, darkest place, and in pain physically, mentally and emotionally, your WHY is what will ground you. No matter what. In times like these, your WHY can make all the difference to make the choice to not give up on your life!

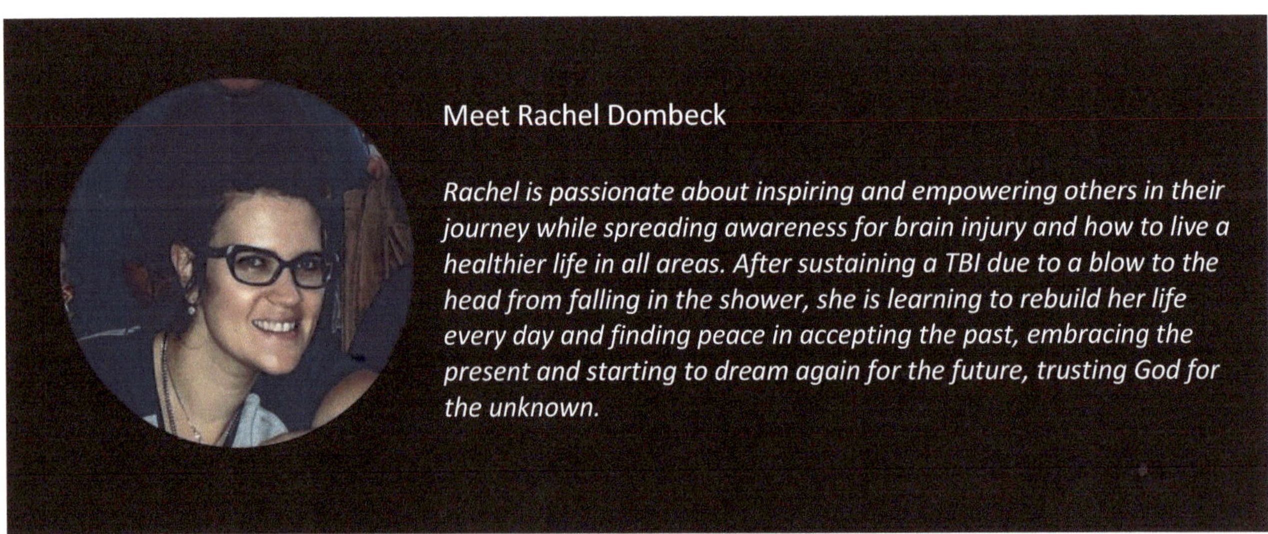

Meet Rachel Dombeck

Rachel is passionate about inspiring and empowering others in their journey while spreading awareness for brain injury and how to live a healthier life in all areas. After sustaining a TBI due to a blow to the head from falling in the shower, she is learning to rebuild her life every day and finding peace in accepting the past, embracing the present and starting to dream again for the future, trusting God for the unknown.

SYMPTOMS OF CONCUSSION

 **PERSONS OF ALL AGES**

"I just don't feel like myself."

Most people with a concussion have one or more of the symptoms listed below and recover fully within days, weeks or a few months. But for some people, symptoms of concussion can last even longer. Generally, if you feel that "something is not quite right," or if you are feeling "foggy," you should talk with your doctor.

Concussion symptoms are often grouped into four categories, including:

THINKING/ REMEMBERING	PHYSICAL	EMOTIONAL/ MOOD	SLEEP DISTURBANCE
• Difficulty thinking clearly • Feeling slowed down • Difficulty concentrating • Difficulty remembering new information	• Headache • Nausea or vomiting (early on) • Balance problems • Dizziness • Fuzzy or blurry vision • Feeling tired, having no energy • Sensitivity to noise or light	• Irritability • Sadness • More emotional • Nervousness or anxiety	• Sleeping more than usual • Sleeping less than usual • Trouble falling asleep

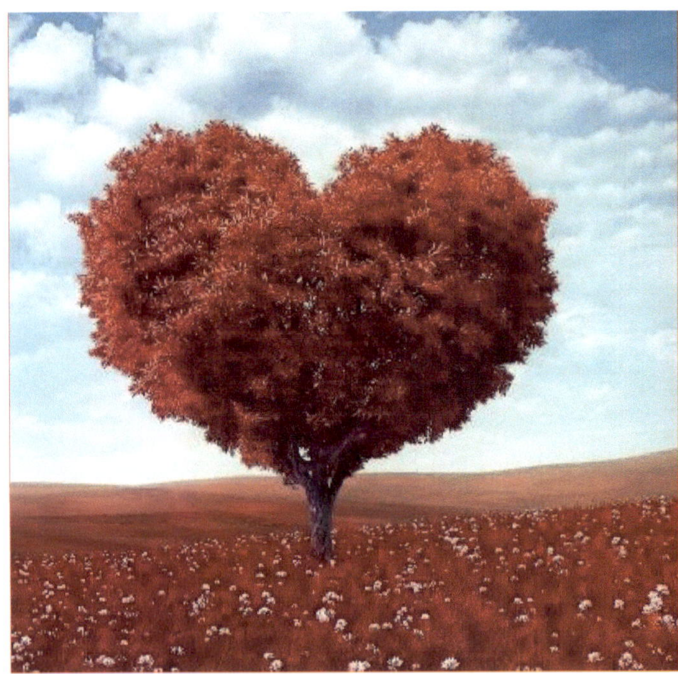

I Am Blessed
By Debra Gorman

According to the magazine Psychology Today, eighty percent of marriages separate by the ten-month mark after brain injury. Statistics also show that over seventy-five percent of marriages plagued by chronic illness end in divorce.

The divorce rate is not a lot better for physically healthy couples, about fifty percent the last time I checked. What makes some couples successful, and others, not so much? I'm sure there are many factors, but I believe it often has to do with the way the two people treat each other.

John and I married in 2005, nearly fourteen years ago. I was fifty years old and he was about to turn fifty. We had both been married before. I felt that I had learned a lot about how *not* to be married and was ready to get it right. We fell passionately, head-over-heels in love and married after dating for two years. We had a fairy tale early marriage.

Additionally, John had recently met a career goal and I was beginning a new profession. Times were good. We continued to enjoy long distance biking, hiking and running. Once I picked the wrong color for the living room. I tried living with it, but when I felt I couldn't, John helped me repaint it with hardly a complaint. His career took us from New York State to Iowa, which was fine with me; a nurse can usually find work easily. Besides, I would have followed him anywhere.

"We had been in Iowa just over a year when, out of the blue, with no warning symptoms, I suffered a brain hemorrhage."

We had been in Iowa just over a year when, out of the blue, with no warning symptoms, I suffered a brain hemorrhage. My condition was precarious in the immediate days and weeks. However, I did rally and after a month I was home, never to be the same person again.

At no time has John ever admitted to me that he was sorry he married me, but it was a concern of mine early on. We had only been married six years and suddenly he was the sole provider and caretaker—although I was fairly independent regarding activities of daily living, albeit extremely clumsy with a loss of balance and coordination.

In the first year I was consumed by sadness and grief over the circumstances in which I found myself. There were so many losses. I worked hard for improvement, but improved very little. Eventually, after many months, I decided to salvage what I could of my life and face forward. I met someone at this time who would become important to me. Beth entered my life as a minister, of sorts, and has since become a lifelong friend.

Other research indicates that men and women need different things from relationships. Women desire love while men crave respect. From my experience I believe that to be true. This is not to say we all don't need both of those things in plentiful supply, just that there is a gender bias that

generally leaves us predisposed to feeling empty without regular demonstrations of one over the other. I am blessed to be told many times each day that I am loved and appreciated. Moreover, John demonstrates his willingness to give me what I need as a person and a wife. In turn, I tell him often how much I respect him and appreciate all he does for us and for me. I also do what I can to demonstrate my feelings. I attempt to make our home a refuge, a place of nurture, rest, and encouragement.

I think these are useful lessons no matter what lifestyle or life stage one is currently in. One need not be married to show love and respect. However, it is beneficial to individual happiness and satisfaction with life to be less consumed by personal interests to concentrate more on affirmation, gratitude, and sharing, in whatever form that may take.

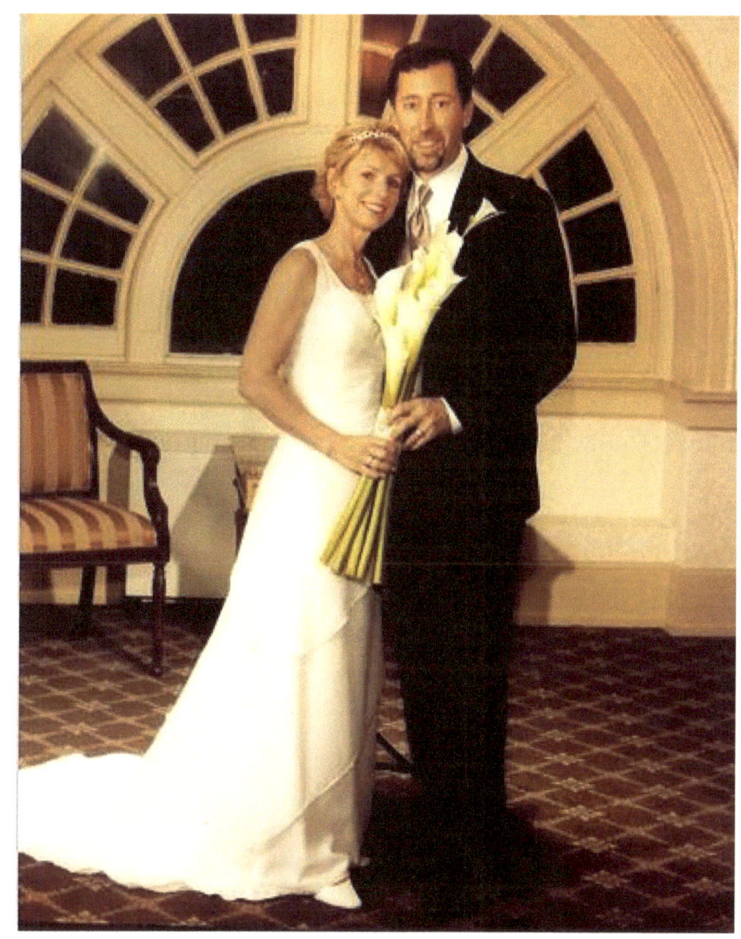

It is unfortunate that I needed to be in my fifties to understand these important life principles. I had always celebrated my abilities but complained that I didn't know my true purpose in life. My interests were so scattered and varied, I couldn't focus effectively. Now, most of those abilities have turned into inabilities. No more long distance running, biking and hiking. No more nursing, and I can no longer execute my decorating schemes because I don't have enough use of my dominant hand. Think about it, what can really be accomplished with only one hand? Simply signing your name requires that you hold the paper with your non dominant hand to keep it from moving.

I have found a handful of things I can still do. Writing is one and I enjoy it a lot. I write to try to motivate all of us to make the best of this life we have been given, to be the best version of ourselves, the person we were created to be. Also, let's choose love, respect, and positive thoughts. It really is a choice.

I find that now I view things from the distance of age as well as catastrophic illness. Both are great teachers—if one is open to learning.

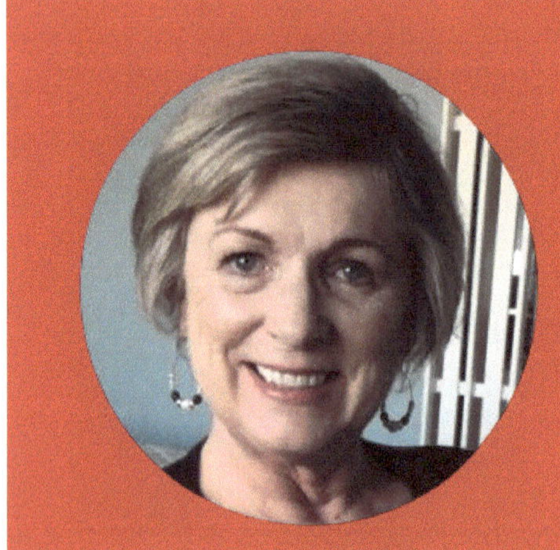

Meet Debra Gorman

Debra Gorman was fifty-six years old in 2011 when she experienced a cavernous angioma on her brain stem, causing her brain to bleed. Four months later she sustained a subdural hematoma. She later learned that she also had suffered a stroke during one of those events. She finds a creative outlet in writing. She enjoys writing for her children and grandchildren and has written articles that have been published for hospice, local newspapers, and Hope magazine. Currently, she writes for her blog, entitled Graceful Journey at debralynn48.wordpress.com.

"Being deeply loved by someone gives you strength, while loving someone deeply gives you courage."

Lao Tzu

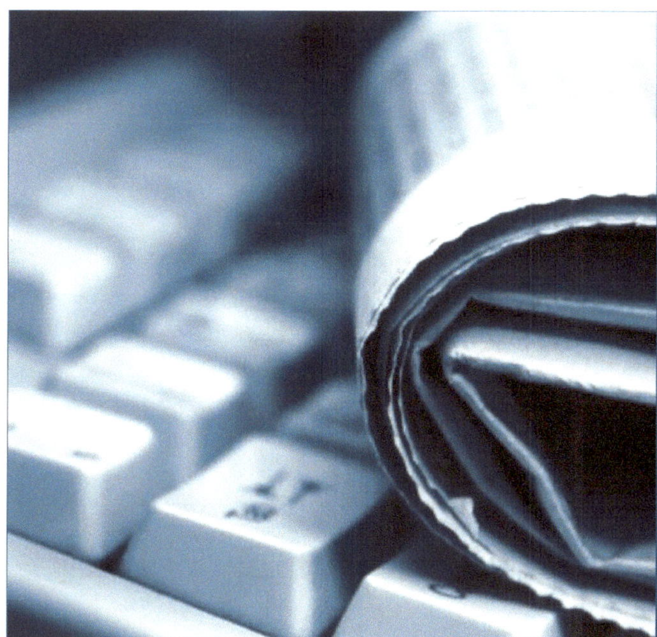

News & Views
David & Sarah Grant

We hope that you've enjoyed this month's issue of HOPE Magazine. Our regular readers no doubt noted our new layout and style. Life, with or without brain injury, is all about change!

On that same note, we are always looking forward, eyes focussed on the horizon, for new and innovative ways to help advocate for those afffected by brain injury. A few years ago, we set our sights on producing a full-length documentary about brain injury. While the idea sounded good, it quickly became clear that we simply did not have several thousand free hours to invest in a project of this magnitude.

Though things are better than they were when brain injury became part of our family, there is still a giant void in brain injury awareness by the general public. Take a random survey and we suspect that you would find that most people have no idea that every year millions of people worldwide are affected by brain injury. The question we have been asking ourselves for many years remains the same, "How can we reach the largest number of people?"

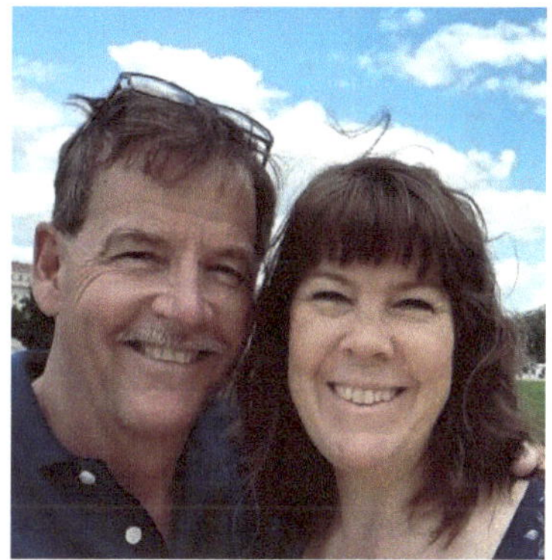

There will be changes coming in 2020. We'll let you in on a little secret! One of the our hopes for next year is to roll out a rather extensive media blitz in the form of short sharable videos. Posted and sharable on a wide range of social platforms, these short videos will be a perfect match for how today's world interfaces with internet content.

And from a creative standpoint, it will give us the opportunity to try something heretofore not done. We are rather fond of being trailblazers!

Until next month,

~ David & Sarah